God's Pathway
to Healing

MENOPAUSE

BOOKS BY
REGINALD B. CHERRY, M.D.

God's Pathway to Healing,
Menopause

God's Pathway to Healing,
Herbs that Heal

God's Pathway to Healing,
Prostate

God's Pathway to Healing

MENOPAUSE

by
Reginald B. Cherry, M.D.
Linda D. Cherry

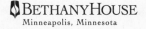

BETHANYHOUSE

Minneapolis, Minnesota

Published by Bethany House Publishers
A Ministry of Bethany Fellowship International
11400 Hampshire Avenue South
Bloomington, Minnesota 55438
www.bethanyhouse.com

Printed in the United States of America by
Bethany Press International
Bloomington, Minnesota 55438

ISBN 1–57778–118–X

CONTENTS

INTRODUCTION

Currently there are 40 to 50 million women in the United States who are post-menopausal, and by the year 2010 this number will increase to 60 million. Amazingly, by the year 2015 almost 50 percent of the women in the United States will be menopausal.

Women are beginning to question more frequently the conventional recommendations of hormone replacement therapy for the rest of their lives, which has been traditionally offered by the medical profession. In fact, studies show that only 10 to 20 percent of the women who are prescribed traditional estrogen replacement therapy (ERT) by physicians continue to take their prescription one year after it is given to them.

Another interesting fact is that women in societies ranging from Latin America to the Mediterranean to Asia seldom experience the problems and menopausal symptoms that women in Western countries experience. The common hot flashes, sweats, mood changes, and so on are encountered very rarely in their societies. Yet if they move to a country such as the United States and follow our typical Western eating habits, they begin to experience the same type of symptoms American women experience.

We are beginning to see the reality of Exodus 23 and the fact that God does truly bless certain foods. As we follow His plan, disease is indeed taken away.

In this mini-book, we will explore *God's Pathway to Healing Menopause*. God's

Word reveals an alternative approach to deal with menopause. We must keep in mind an incredible revelation: *God provided estrogen in the plant kingdom for women to use as their ovaries cease producing it.*

Remarkably, over 300 different plants that contain estrogen have been identified. The goals of medical professionals like ourselves who believe in an alternative approach to traditional estrogen therapy are:

- To provide women relief from the common menopausal symptoms (hot flashes, sweats, etc.)

- To prevent bone thinning (osteoporosis), heart disease, skin changes, and hair loss

- To eliminate or significantly reduce the incidence of Alzheimer's disease and colon cancer

- To help prevent breast and uterine cancer

We believe there is a Pathway to Healing for lessening or eliminating many of the uncomfortable and painful symptoms women often experience during menopause. If you are a woman in this time of life, or know a woman who is, this minibook is packed with information that will help uncover God's unique *Pathway to Healing* for you.

Reginald B. Cherry, M.D.

Linda D. Cherry

Chapter 1

GOD HAS A PATHWAY
TO HEALING FOR YOU

Chapter 1

GOD HAS A PATHWAY TO HEALING FOR YOU

The understanding of healing can be very complex and very frustrating. As we walk through this world, we face the constant attacks from the forces of darkness. Jesus made it clear that we have an enemy who is out "to steal, and to kill, and to destroy" (John 10:10). The enemy is not as interested in attacking our physical bodies as much as hindering the anointing that is contained *within* our physical bodies.

Second Corinthians 4:7 says, "But we have this treasure in earthen vessels, that the excellency of the power may be of God, and not of us." This treasure is the anointing power of God that resides within us. It is for this reason that the enemy is so intent on trying to cripple and weaken our bodies — so that he can stop the anointing that resides within.

One of the first things we like to point out to patients is that we were actually healed 2,000 years ago through the blood of Jesus. First Peter 2:24 tells us that we *were* healed by the stripes of Jesus. This scripture gives us a great insight into healing and how we should view it.

Since we were healed 2,000 years ago, what we are actually seeking and believing God for is the *manifestation* of healing in our bodies. It may seem like a minor point, but when you begin praying for God to illuminate the pathway that will lead to the manifestation of healing in your body, you are "rightly dividing the word" (2 Timothy 2:15). You are acknowledging before God the incredible sacrifice He made by placing our disease and infirmity upon the body of His own precious Son. Jesus bore in His body not only the sins of man, but also the diseases of man which are the result of sin.

Now let's take two simple illustrations from two different healings recorded during Jesus' ministry. We want you to consider two scriptures, Mark 10:46 and John 9:4-7. The revelations contained in these two healings Jesus performed literally changed the way we practice medicine.

In these two scriptures we see two men, each with the same disease (blindness), each having an encounter with Jesus, and each being totally healed. From the time of their encounter with Jesus until healing was manifested in their bodies, however, we see a totally different set of circumstances.

As we examine these two healings, we want you to understand that there is a unique pathway to your healing from the symptoms and potentially serious diseases associated with menopause. It was never God's intent or will for you to suffer in your body as natural hormonal changes take place, so be encouraged as we discover God's healing pathway for you.

HEALING MAY MANIFEST SUPERNATURALLY

Many of the healings of Jesus occurred instantly, supernaturally, and dramatically, while at other times healing was a process. For example, in Luke 17:14 the ten lepers were healed "as they went." In the case of Bartimaeus, Mark 10:46-52, we see two important principles at work:

1. Express your faith that the Lord can and will heal. In His encounter with Bartimaeus, Jesus knew his affliction but nevertheless asked him, "What wilt thou that I should do unto thee?" He asked Bartimaeus this question in order to get the blind man to express his faith by telling Jesus, "that I might receive my sight."

2. Speak to the mountain of your affliction. Bartimaeus spoke directly to the problem — his blindness. He expressed his faith that the Lord would heal his blindness. It was Bartimaeus' faith that made him whole, and he received an immediate and complete manifestation of his healing from blindness.

YOUR PATHWAY TO HEALING MAY INVOLVE A PROCESS

Now let's compare the healing of Bartimaeus with the healing that occurred in John 9:1-7. This is perhaps one of the most unusual healings recorded in Jesus' ministry. Nevertheless, it is recorded in the Word of God to give us a unique revelation on healing.

Remember, this man had the same disease as Bartimaeus; that is, he was blind. When Jesus touched him and anointed his eyes with a mixture of mud and saliva, interestingly, there was not an instant manifestation of healing. In fact, Jesus gave the man a set of instructions, directing him to go down a pathway, reach down into the pool called Siloam, place water in his hands, and wash his eyes.

Why, of all of the healings Jesus performed, was this one included in the Bible? The key part of this account is found in John 9:7 where it states, "He went his way therefore, and washed, and came seeing." We believe it illustrates two important revelations about healing.

1. The manifestation of your healing may involve your following a set of instructions, and

2. As you are led by the Holy Spirit and "go your way," you will be healed.

God instructed us to teach people that they too have a unique *Pathway to Healing.* We see in this scripture that healing anointing can flow through natural substances; that is, substances we can touch, taste, feel, and so on. In this case, the healing anointing from Jesus flowed through mud and saliva.

As we study the Bible, we see from Genesis to Revelation the emphasis that God has placed on natural substances, and that He uses them to bring about the manifestation of our healing. We see how plants, certain animals, and the leaves of trees (see Revelation 22:2) were used as part of the Pathway to Healing for man.

As we review Mark 10 and John 9 and the healings that are illustrated, we can petition God to reveal to each of us our unique Pathway to Healing through the leading of the Holy Spirit — the One who guides us into all truth and shows us things to come. Often in the healings we see with our patients, the Pathway to Healing involves a combination of both reliance on supernatural intervention and the use of natural substances.

By understanding these two illustrations from Jesus' ministry and seeking God for our Pathway to Healing, we are not limiting God. We are being totally open in our petitions to Him by acknowledging Him as the supernatural Healer and also acknowledging that He provided natural ways through which healing anointing may flow!

YOU HAVE A PATHWAY TO HEALING FOR THE SYMPTOMS OF MENOPAUSE

As we begin to explore the specific ways God provided to help women through menopause and protect them from the devastating diseases that occur during this period in a woman's life, constantly and continually remind yourself of the examples of healing with the two blind men. Realize the supernatural power of healing that God has provided as you speak to the mountain (see Mark 11:23) — the hot flashes, the sweats, the mood changes, and the other problems of menopause.

Your faith in God will increase as you study these scriptures, for it is faith that gives "the substance of things hoped for" (Hebrews 11:1). You will also realize that it is not the natural substances in and of themselves that heal, but it is God's anointing that flows through those natural substances that brings the manifestation of healing. It is the power of God that literally holds the molecules of every natural substance together. (See Colossians 1:17.)

God has provided you with ways to pray specifically and with understanding for menopause. Your pathway may involve a combination of supernatural healing, the use of natural substances, speaking to the mountain of symptoms, and above all, exercising your faith in God.

The price for your healing has already been paid! So now let's seek together some insights God has given so that we can be set free from the symptoms and diseases associated with menopause.

Chapter 2

GOD'S PATHWAY
TO HEALING
MENOPAUSE

Chapter 2

GOD'S PATHWAY TO HEALING MENOPAUSE

What are the signs and symptoms of menopause? As a woman nears the end of her childbearing years, at first the ovaries begin to secrete hormones erratically. This is termed the "perimenopause." During this time in her life (which can begin as early as the late 30s, though it is more typically seen in the mid 40s) periods may be somewhat irregular; that is, they may be shortened or lengthened. She may begin having hot flashes and sweats.

PERIMENOPAUSE

The phase prior to the onset of menopause, during which the woman with regular menses changes, perhaps abruptly, to a pattern of irregular cycles and increased periods of amenorrhea. For epidemiological investigations, the inception of perimenopause is characterized by 3 to 11 months of amenorrhea or, for those without amenorrhea, increased menstrual irregularity. While menopause has a clear and accepted definition, perimenopause does not.

(Taber's Cyclopedic Medical Dictionary, 1997)

Women may continue to have regular periods each month, but they also may begin having some of the typical menopausal symptoms. The ovaries begin to produce lower and lower hormone levels and the adrenal glands and fatty tissue in a woman's body take over the production of estrogen, though in much lesser amounts.

What Is Menopause

Menopause is defined as the loss of ovarian function which is characterized by the cessation of menstrual periods. Estrogen and progesterone levels decline dramatically and the FSH and LH chemical levels in the blood increase. It is at this time that women often experience the traditional symptoms of menopause, such as hot flashes, sweats, mood changes, and so on.

MENOPAUSE

The period that marks the permanent cessation of menstrual activity, usually occurring between the ages of 35 and 58. The menses may stop suddenly, there may be a decreased flow each month until a final cessation, or the interval between periods may be lengthened until complete cessation is accomplished. Natural menopause will occur in 25 percent of women by age 47, in 50 percent by age 50, 75 percent by age 52, and in 95 percent by age 55. Menopause due to surgical removal of the ovaries has occurred in almost 30 percent of U.S. women who are 50 years of age or older. Women with short menstrual cycles may reach menopause as much as two years earlier than women with long cycles. Cigarette smoking has an effect on menopause, causing it to occur 1 to 2 years prematurely.

(Taber's Cyclopedic Medical Dictionary, 1997)

THE MENOPAUSE CHECKLIST

Are you approaching menopause or have you already arrived at this point in your life? Check any of the symptoms listed below that you may be experiencing now. If you are having three or more of these symptoms, you may well be entering into menopause:

__ Dry skin, dry hair, or vaginal dryness

__ Irregular menstrual periods

__ Increased irritability and mood swings

__ Pain with intercourse

__ Increased symptoms of anxiety, nervousness, and depression

__ Increased craving for sweets and sudden binge eating

__ Sudden hot flashes

__ Decreased mental alertness

__ Difficulty sleeping

__ Vaginal pain or itching

__ Loss of skin tone, hair loss, or increased bruising

__ Breast tenderness

__ Low back pain or pain in the hip area

__ Abnormal hair growth above the lip

If three or more of these symptoms fit your physical condition, you should consult with a knowledgeable physician to discuss treatment for menopause.

Does God have a plan to protect women during and after menopause, and have we simply ignored it? Is there a way to avoid or significantly lessen the symptoms mentioned above? Is there something in the diet of Asian women that we lack? I believe God is trying to reveal something to us that we are just now beginning to understand.

The menopausal era of a woman's life not only produces the annoying symptoms described, but can increase dramatically the risk of serious disease, especially heart attacks and bone thinning leading to osteoporosis, broken hips, etc. In fact, by the age of 65, women have as many heart attacks as men due to the lack of estrogen produced.

Doctors have traditionally prescribed a conjugated estrogen such as *Premarin,* which indeed protects women from heart disease and other symptoms, but causes an increase in breast and uterine cancer. The real advantage of the more natural methods, using plant-derived estrogens (which are phenolic estrogens) is that they provide the same benefits of the conjugated estrogens (preventing hot flashes, protecting from heart disease, etc.) but actually protect women from breast and uterine cancer.

Isn't it amazing that within the plant kingdom God has placed numerous estrogen-like hormones which only recently have come to light through medical research? Why would He do this?

The answer to this question and our understanding of plant hormones can benefit the lives of millions of women (and even men) which we shall explore later. Some of the greatest medical challenges facing modern medicine are the direct result of hormone levels decreasing as women grow older.

It is this drop in a woman's natural production of estrogen during menopause and perimenopause that results in the dreaded menopausal symptoms of hot flashes, sweats, mood swings, forgetfulness, sleep problems, and bones becoming brittle.

Even more ominous is the steady increase in heart attacks, strokes, diabetes, and Alzheimer's disease as a woman's ovaries begin to shut down, not to mention the increased risk of breast cancer. God has already made a provision to protect women from these problems, as we will soon discuss.

THE TRADITIONAL APPROACH — PREMARIN

As women live longer, the rate of breast and ovarian cancer rises alarmingly. Doctors do their best to help women by prescribing various hormones, the most common being *Premarin,* which comes from the urine of pregnant mares.

Premarin helps alleviate hot flashes and decreases the rate of heart attacks, but it has a dark side: it can increase the risk of breast and ovarian cancer, can cause bloating and weight gain, and must be taken the rest of a woman's life. Surely there must be a better way!

Did God intend for women to give birth to children the first half of their lives and then spend the last of their days suffering the ravages of disease because their ovaries quit producing estrogen? God said in Psalm 91:16, "With long life will I sat-isfy him, and shew him my salvation."

God's Pathway to Healing for us includes living a long, satisfied life. Hot flashes, breast cancer, broken hips, stooped backs with collapsed vertebrae, heart attacks, and other ailments are definitely not fulfilling God's promise in Psalm 91. These do not represent a "satisfied" long life!

WHY IS IT THAT ASIAN WOMEN DON'T SUFFER DURING MENOPAUSE?

Here's another question we need to address: Why is it that women in Asia, as well as certain Latin American countries and Mediterranean countries, go through menopause but don't have the hot flashes, sweats, mood changes, broken bones, etc. that women in the United States have — nor do they have any significant problem with breast cancer and heart disease? Yet when these same women move to the United States, they begin having the typical menopausal symptoms women in America have!

PLANT-DERIVED ESTROGENS

Research is beginning to shed light on God's plan to take care of women. The evidence is pointing to substances found in foods, especially a group of substances known as *phytoestrogens* (plant-derived estrogens). God has created phytoestrogens as part of our Pathway to Healing.

During the course of a woman's life, from teen years until menopause, a woman's ovaries produce what are known as *steroidal* estrogens. This type of estrogen causes the ovaries to produce eggs and enables a woman to have children.

However, the story gets more complicated. Though the steroidal estrogens are essential for reproduction and protect a woman from heart disease, osteoporosis, hair thinning, and numerous other problems, they also have a dark side. Here are some examples:

1. The longer a woman is exposed to naturally produced estrogen, the greater the risk she will have in her later years of breast cancer and ovarian cancer. It is the length of time the female body is exposed to estrogen that increases the risk of cancer later.

2. Breast cancer is higher in women who begin having periods earlier and enter menopause later in life.

3. It has also been noted that breast cancer occurs less in women who have more children, because during pregnancy estrogen production ceases.

So the risk of cancer is only compounded when a doctor prescribes a steroidal estrogen like *Premarin* when women go through menopause. When doctors prescribe *Premarin,* they may help make a woman feel better after menopause and even reduce her risk of some diseases, but the trade off is this: her cancer risk is increased by continuing steroidal-type estrogen longer than God intended.

GOD'S NATURAL PATHWAY

What if we could alleviate a woman's menopausal symptoms, such as hot flashes, sweats, and memory changes; and protect her from heart disease, osteoporosis, and breast, uterine, and ovarian cancer? That sounds like the way God would do it. This is becoming a very intriguing story, isn't it?

Let's turn our attention back to the plant kingdom. God said He would "bless thy bread, and thy water; and I will take sickness away from the midst of thee"

(Exodus 23:25). God also stated in Revelation 22:2 that "the leaves of the tree were for the healing of the nations."

Earlier in this chapter, we mentioned phytoestrogens. God created plants with estrogen compounds. But these "plant estrogens" are different from the body's own estrogens and are different from the estrogens doctors commonly prescribe. They are known as *phenolic estrogens.* It is these kinds of estrogens, which we mentioned earlier, that women in Asia and Latin America consume daily in their normal diets.

What is different about these plant estrogens? Plant or phenolic estrogens can attach to receptors for certain organs of the body, such as the breasts and uterus. They actually modulate or block the effect of a woman's own estrogen on these tissues. The bottom line is that plant estrogens created by God can protect a woman from breast, ovarian, and uterine cancer in her later years!

This is probably a major reason breast cancer, for example, is so low in Asia and parts of Latin America — people of these nations consume phyto (phenolic) estrogens in their foods most of their lives.

So what happens when Asian women go through menopause? The plant estrogens take over after their ovaries shut down and keep them from having the usual hot flashes, sweats, and other menopausal symptoms while protecting them from the most common female cancers. It sounds almost too good to be true, but God's plan always is, isn't it?

Now we will explore the foods you need to eat in order to take care of your temple — your body (see 1 Corinthians 6:19) — during and after menopause.

Chapter 3

GOOD NUTRITION
DURING AND
AFTER MENOPAUSE

Chapter 3

GOOD NUTRITION
DURING AND
AFTER MENOPAUSE

What are Asian women eating that
keeps them from experiencing menopausal
symptoms or having breast cancer? They
are eating according to Genesis 1:29!

"And God said, Behold, I have
given you every herb bearing seed,
which is upon the face of all the
earth, and every tree, in the which
is the fruit of a tree yielding seed;
to you it shall be for meat."

Estrogen occurs throughout the plant kingdom, and you would have to be on a plant-free diet to avoid it. Five major types of phytoestrogens have been identified:

1. Flavanones (citrus fruit)
2. Isoflavones (legumes, such as chickpeas, soy, lentils, clover, and beans)
3. Flavonols (red and yellow fruit and vegetables)
4. Flavones (red and yellow fruit and vegetables)
5. Lignans (flaxseed and cereals)

Most plants contain several different types of estrogen. Certain herbs like black cohosh and the roots of some plants like licorice also contain estrogenic compounds. However, the highest estrogen activity is found in the isoflavone group (the legumes) and it is the legume diet that is so widely consumed in Asian, Latin American, and Mediterranean countries.

The highest natural estrogen levels are found in soy-based foods (tofu, miso), kidney beans, lima beans, and chickpeas.

There are four major isoflavones: genistein, daidzein, biochanin, and formononetin. These protective compounds come mainly from certain plants, and these foods can become a major source in your nutrition to help protect you from breast cancer and some of the uncomfortable symptoms of menopause.

FOODS THAT CONTAIN PLANT ISOFLAVONES

- split peas
- kidney beans
- lima beans
- chickpeas
- soy products like tofu and miso

Here is the amazing thing: *the women in the countries mentioned above consume 30-*

50 mg. of isoflavones daily. In this country we average 2-4 mg. daily! We are just beginning to understand what God created to protect us.

Researchers are currently studying a group of prescription drugs known as SERMs (selective estrogen receptor modulators). These are actually "antiestrogen" compounds that block the detrimental effects of estrogen and are used to treat, and possibly prevent, breast cancer and osteoporosis. *Tamoxifen* and *Raloxifene* are the first two available, but unfortunately they have some significant side effects.

God has already been there ahead of us. The phytoestrogens are the original SERMs, which can protect us from breast cancer and, more importantly, have none of the side effects the prescription medicines have. God has even given scientists the wisdom to know how to isolate these major plant estrogens in a nonprescription tablet (but more on that later).

FOODS TO ADD TO YOUR DIET

Perhaps the food product that should be emphasized the most would be soy. The phytoestrogens (plant-derived estrogens) contained in soy products are isoflavones. Studies now demonstrate that these products from soy decrease hot flashes, vaginal dryness and thinning, as well as bone loss, the risk of uterine cancer, and probably help prevent colon cancer.

There are many ways to obtain soy products (tofu, miso, etc.) but many of these are difficult for those in Western countries to consume and prepare, simply because they are unfamiliar to us. We are recommending to our patients that they consider products such as soy milk. This is available at health food stores and other specialty stores and is often formulated as low calorie milk shakes. The taste of soy milk can be enhanced by adding almond extract to it, which is very effective in improving the taste (if that's a problem for you).

Another option is to use soy protein powder. At M.D. Anderson Cancer Center in Houston, doctors counsel their patients to use soy protein in the form of soy protein isolate powder. Another option is to obtain a cereal known as Nutlettes. This is a breakfast cereal which is crunchy and very similar to Grape Nuts, but it has a very high content of isoflavones from soy.

Isoflavones are metabolized (broken down) in the gut, and adding yogurt with live cultures of acidophilus or lactobacillus will enhance the absorption of the estrogen compounds in the blood.

It is also beneficial for women to use a high-fiber cereal, such as 1/3 to 1/2 cup of

FiberOne or 1/3 cup of oat bran, as this helps prevent some of the more toxic by-products of naturally produced estrogen from being reabsorbed into the blood stream through the colon.

Another beneficial food product is flaxseed, and flaxseeds actually are better than flaxseed oil. This contains phyto-estrogens known as lignans. These, similar to soy products, are acted upon by colonic bacteria to produce certain forms of estrogen which are very safe and absorbed into the blood stream. They too can offer protection against breast cancer by binding to estrogen sites in the breast and in the tissue lining the uterus.

It is also beneficial to eat more of the coldwater fish, particularly salmon, cod, and herring, because of the omega-3 fatty acids (natural essential fatty acids found prominently in foods such as certain fish) that prevent heart disease, the major killer of women.

Exercise, such as simply walking three miles in 45-50 minutes three days weekly, will decrease circulating estrogen levels the body produces, help prevent osteoporosis, lower blood pressure, and protect the heart and blood vessels.

To summarize the dietary staples of God's pathway to combating the common symptoms associated with menopause:

Soy Milk. A good source of natural estrogen is soy milk, 8-12 ounces daily, or soy protein that can be mixed in with other foods. There are many ways to add soy to your nutritional intake, such as adding soy milk to cereal, substituting soy milk for cow's milk when you cook, using soy cheese, and trying soy protein to substitute at times in your diet for animal protein.

Tofu and miso. Tofu and miso are other traditional soy products that can be added to the diet. The pale, spongy texture of tofu is difficult for many people to consume. However, the advantage of tofu is that it takes on the flavor of whatever it is cooked with and can be used in meats, soups, vegetables, and dessert dishes.

Legumes. Adding daily servings of legumes, such as lima beans, kidney beans, split peas, or lentils will also dramatically increase phytoestrogen levels in the blood.

Recent studies have shown that soy isoflavones increase bone mineral density and can prevent, and perhaps reverse, osteoporosis. A high soy diet can decrease the risk of breast cancer in women and prostate cancer in men, two of our most common cancers. In men the plant-derived estrogens offset the negative effects of the male hormone testosterone. Asian men seldom get prostate cancer because of their high soy diet. Diets rich in beans can reduce uterine cancer rates as well.

Black cohosh. Black cohosh is a plant containing phytoestrogens and has produced an 80 percent improvement in menopausal symptoms, such as hot flashes, headaches, depression, and heart palpitations. This is now available as an over-the-counter supplement. We recommend a dose of 80 mg. daily.

Flaxseed. A class of chemical compounds known as lignans can also produce the benefits associated with the isoflavones (such as found in soy products). Flaxseed is a popular source.

Many herbs contain phytoestrogens, such as chasteberry, anise, dong quai, ginseng, sage, red clover, licorice root, etc. Other plants containing phytoestrogens include licorice root, oats, almonds, apples, alfalfa, cashews, peanuts, and wheat.

Daily intake of phytoestrogens is essential. These plant-derived estrogens improve mood, ease sleeping patterns, and relieve hot flashes. They have the added benefit of protecting women from breast and uterine cancer and also offer protection from heart disease, osteoporosis, and even Alzheimer's disease.

In some women, because of unique risk factors for cardiovascular disease or other unique individual situations, a prescription estrogen product is needed. We are not prescribing the traditional estrogen *Premarin* (which is used by over 80 percent of traditional medical doctors) but instead use safer, "friendlier" estrogens such as Estrace (beta-estradiol) or Ogen (estrone sulfate).

With these products, you will need a supplemental progesterone to protect from uterine cancer. Women with a hysterectomy do not need to add progesterone, but they may benefit from it for other symptoms. Here, again, the trend is away from traditional synthetic progestins such as *Provera*. We are now using *Prometrium*, which is a natural micronized progesterone. Other options for estrogen replacement therapy include the use of the compounded tri-estrogen (estriol, estrone, and beta-estradiol).

We would suggest consulting with a doctor (hopefully one familiar with the newer plant-derived products and safer estrogens) before beginning treatment on your own. We often try the natural plant-derived products as our first approach. We have been seeing some of the best results with the new plant with the new plant-derived capsule, *Menopause Support* which will be discussed later in this chapter.

MANAGING YOUR
MENOPAUSAL SYMPTOMS

Female patients often complain that the most uncomfortable symptom of menopause is the hot flash, which starts suddenly as a warmth in the face, head, or chest. In just moments, a hot flash can spread throughout a woman's body. As the body tries to cool itself, she begins sweating and her body may react with a bout of shivering chills, which results from wide-open pores and damp skin.

We have some basic recommendations for managing menopause with supplements. We recommend 1,500 mg. of calcium, such as calcium carbonate or calcium citrate (always take with food).

Our usual recommendations of the various antioxidants and multivitamins are also very helpful, and studies have shown that vitamin E (400-800 I.U.) can help prevent some of the hot flashes associated with menopause. Remember that it may take a few weeks for vitamin E to become effective.

There are many herbal-type formulations available, such as *Menopause Support,* which contain all four of the basic isoflavones. We will discuss this later.

Because mood changes and depression are so common with menopause, we sometimes use St. John's Wort 0.3 percent 300 mg. three times daily. Ginkgo biloba is also used to help increase blood flow to the brain and help with memory disturbances.

In summary, menopausal symptoms can be managed with these supplements:

Calcium – 1,500 mg. daily. The National Institutes of Health recommend that women in their childbearing years get at least 1,000 mg. of calcium a day. But past menopause, the recommendation is 1,500 mg. Ways to get plenty of calcium in your diet include: 1 cup of skim milk (320 mg. of calcium or 30 percent of the DV); an 8 oz. serving of yogurt (415 mg. of calcium or 41 percent of the DV); and 3 oz. of salmon, which has 181 mg. of calcium (18 percent of the DV).

Vitamin E — 400-800 I.U. daily.

Valerian — 2.5-5.0 mg. for sleep.

Gingko can help with memory changes (40 mg. 2-3 times daily).

St. John's Wort has been shown to be useful for depression and mood changes (0.3 percent, 300 mg., three times daily).

For more information about vitamins and antioxidants, see the Appendix at the end of this book.

Many of these vitamins and minerals are contained in the Mediterranean diet which we have described for you at the end of this chapter.

PHYTOESTROGENS: *A RECENT MEDICAL BREAKTHROUGH*

There are now many natural hormones that are available in tablet and capsule form. For example, there are tablets of isoflavones, which are available at health food stores. We have been getting some almost miraculous stories from women who have been taking a product called *Promensil,* which we have discussed in the past on our weekly television program.

Promensil is a basic formulation that contains four of the isoflavones. It is a dietary plant estrogen available over the counter. The typical dose is one or two tablets daily, but many women require up to four per day because of varying levels of absorption.

A more complete formulation is now available in a product called *Menopause Support. Menopause Support* is a unique and comprehensive natural dietary supplement that I have formulated personally, based on my 25 years of research and medical practice. It contains a combination of the seven minerals, herbs, and plant extracts that I personally recommend. The typical dose is two capsules daily. (See back of this book for order information.)

Remember, taking a natural supplement like this is very much like switching to the Asian or Mediterranean diet, and it should really not be looked upon as a medication, but rather a plant-derived product. It is very safe and does not require a progesterone supplement (as do many of the prescription estrogens) if you still have your uterus. It can also be used if you have been diagnosed with or have a history of breast cancer.

Women usually begin noticing benefits in four to six weeks after beginning this pill, but if you are not feeling the effects after six weeks, the dosage should be increased. If you are already on a prescription medicine, allow up to six weeks of taking both *Menopause Support* and the prescription medicine before decreasing the prescription medication.

We recommend a dose of two capsules daily. Remember that you should try it for 12 weeks to see if it will benefit you in regard to menopausal symptoms.

Even if you are not having symptoms of menopause, studies show *Menopause Support* will help provide long-term protection from breast cancer, heart disease, and osteoporosis.

THE MEDITERRANEAN DIET

The Mediterranean diet contains many of the food sources rich in the vitamins and minerals needed for consumption for women during and after menopause. This diet closely corresponds to Genesis 1:29 and 9:3. We highly recommend this diet.

1. Olive oil. Replaces most fats, oils, butter, and margarine. Use in salads or cook with it. Raises levels of the good cholesterol (HDL) and may strengthen immune system functions. Extra virgin olive oil is preferable.

2. Bread. Consume daily, not sliced white bread or even sliced wheat bread, but either make or buy dark, chewy, crusty loaves.

3. Pasta, Rice, Couscous, Bulgur, and Potatoes. Pasta is often served with fresh vegetables and herbs sautéed in olive oil, occasionally with small quantities of lean beef. Dark rice is preferred. Couscous and bulgur are forms of wheat.

4. Grains. Alternate cereals such as wheat bran, 1/2 cup, 4-5 times weekly, and Bran Buds (1/2 cup) or oat bran (1/3 cup).

5. Fruit. Preferably raw, 2-3 pieces daily.

6. Beans. Pintos, great northern, navy, kidney, 1/2 cup, 3-4 times weekly. Bean and lentil soups are very popular (with a small amount of olive oil). Remember that beans are legumes which are filled with phytoestrogens.

7. Nuts. Almonds (10 per day) or walnuts (10 per day) are at the top of the list.

8. Vegetables. Dark green vegetables are prominent, especially in salads. Eat at least one of these daily (cabbage, broccoli, cauliflower, turnip greens, or mustard greens) and one of these daily (carrots, spinach, sweet potatoes, cantaloupe, peaches, or apricots).

9. Cheese and Yogurt. Unlike milk and milk products, some recent studies indicate cheese may not contribute as much to clogged arteries. In the Mediterranean diet, cheese may be grated on soups or a small wedge may be combined with a piece of fruit for dessert. Use the reduced-fat varieties (the fat-free often taste like rubber). The best yogurt is fat-free, but not frozen.

You should consume the following foods only a few times weekly:

10. Fish. The healthiest are coldwater varieties: cod, salmon, and mackerel. Trout is also good. All these are high in omega-3 fatty acids. Salmon is an excellent source of calcium, which is so essential to your intake, even more so after menopause.

11. Poultry. Can be eaten 2-3 times weekly. White breast meat is best, and remove skin.

12. Eggs. Eat in small amounts 2-3 times weekly.

Consume the following an average of three times per month:

13. Red Meat. Use only lean cuts with fat trimmed. Also use in small amounts to "spice up" soup or pasta. The severe restriction of red meat in the Mediterranean diet is a radical departure from the American diet and is a major contributor to the low cancer and heart disease rates in these countries.

Typically, a Mediterranean meal would consist of:

1. Salad. Eat with each meal. Fresh greens and other vegetables with olive oil, vinegar, and/or lemon juice.

2. Soup. Often with chopped celery, garlic, carrots, onions (sometimes in a chicken stock), with added herbs and a small amount of grated cheese (use low-fat).

3. Pasta. A staple of many meals, often made with fresh vegetables and herbs sautéed in olive oil, occasionally a bit of beef or chicken is added.

4. Rice. Prominent in this diet and includes dark rice, pilafs, etc.

5. Breakfast: Often dark bread or cereal (such as those mentioned above), a piece of fresh fruit, and perhaps a small amount of yogurt or a slice of cheese.

6. Tomatoes, onions, lemon juice. All common in the Mediterranean diet.

Chapter 4

PRAYING WITH UNDERSTANDING FOR MENOPAUSE

Chapter 4

PRAYING WITH UNDERSTANDING FOR MENOPAUSE

God's Pathway to Healing has six specific principles for identifying your particular Pathway to Healing menopause. Your healing may supernaturally and instantaneously manifest, or you may experience a process that combines His supernatural power with wisdom, taking the specific actions necessary to obtain your healing.

Your Pathway to Healing may involve a passage of time in which you will want to both pray and care for your physical temple — your body.

To know what actions God desires you to take, you need to pray about menopause with understanding. The Bible urges us to pray with understanding: "What is it then? I will pray with the spirit, and I will *pray with the understanding* also" (1 Corinthians 14:15; emphasis ours). To pray with understanding, apply these six principles that will reveal your Pathway to Healing.

PRINCIPLE 1:
CAST YOUR CARES ON THE LORD

Negative, unhealthy, and destructive emotions like fear, anxiety, and worry can hinder your prayers about menopause and keep you from understanding what actions the Holy Spirit wants you to take. First Peter 5:7 AMP states, "Casting the whole of your care — all your anxieties, all your worries, all your concerns, once and for all — on Him; for He cares for you affectionately, and cares about you watchfully."

If you are facing worries and fears about menopause, we want to reassure you that by the stripes of Jesus you have been healed. (See 1 Peter 2:24.) We often share with patients, "You must cast all of your anxieties and cares upon God. Cast your worries upon the Lord once and for all!"

We might have a woman worried about menopause pray these words:

Father, in the name of Jesus I come before Your throne. You instructed me in 1 Peter 5:7 to cast all of my care, all of my worry, and all of my anxiety once and for all upon You, and because You instructed me to do this, I know that I am capable of doing this and being set free of anxiety. So I cast the anxiety I have about heart dis-

ease, broken bones, breast cancer, hot flashes, and all of the symptoms that go along with menopause upon You. You did not give me a spirit of fear, so I cast all of my concern about menopause upon You, and I thank You that, according to Psalm 91, I will be satisfied with long life. Amen.

We will also warn her that the fear is very likely to attack again a day or two after we have prayed. So we tell her not to pray the same prayer about fear again. Instead, we explain that the devil is attacking her mind with fear and she should now declare to him:

Satan, I have cast anxiety about menopause on my heavenly Father, just as He told me to do. He would not tell me to cast my cares upon Him unless it was something I am capable of doing. Therefore, Satan, I take

authority over you, and I command
you to stop attacking my mind with
fearful thoughts.

PRINCIPLE 2:
PRAY AND PETITION GOD FOR
YOUR PATHWAY TO HEALING

Our key text here is Philippians 4:6-7, "But in every thing by prayer and supplication with thanksgiving let your requests be made known unto God. And the peace of God, which passeth all understanding, shall keep your hearts and minds through Christ Jesus." Pray according to these verses:

Father, I thank You that You will
reveal to me the specific pathway that
will lead to my healing of any and all
symptoms related to menopause.

I thank You, Father, that in Jesus'
name I will not experience problems

with hot flashes, sweats, and mood changes.

I thank You, Lord, that as my natural estrogen levels decrease I will not suffer from heart disease, osteoporosis, and Alzheimer's disease.

I thank You, Father, that You have provided ways to protect my temple through the use of plant-derived estrogens. They will protect me not only from the symptoms of menopause, but also from the increased risk of disease that menopause can bring on.

Thank You, Father, for granting these petitions, in Jesus' name. Amen.

PRINCIPLE 3:
TEST YOUR OPTIONS
BY THE SPIRIT OF GOD

As you seek God for your Pathway to Healing menopause, let the Holy Spirit reveal your options and check or stop any choices that He does not desire you to take. The Bible instructs us: "And let the peace (soul harmony which comes) from Christ rule (act as umpire continually) in your hearts [deciding and settling with finality all questions that arise in your minds, in that peaceful state] to which as [members of Christ's] one body you were also called [to live]. And be thankful (appreciative), [giving praise to God always]" (Colossians 3:15 AMP).

The Spirit of God helps us to consider carefully our options — He umpires our choices — until we reach a decision that brings complete peace in our lives. Simply pray:

> *Father, I pray that Your Holy Spirit will be an umpire in my life, guiding me to every right decision in Your will for me. Grant me Your*

peace in each decision that Your Spirit guides me through. In Jesus' name. Amen.

PRINCIPLE 4:
SPEAK TO THE MOUNTAIN

Now you are ready to speak to the mountain. Instead of just praying, petitioning, and testing, you can go even further in your walk with God. Jesus taught us to speak to our mountain and command that illness to be removed.

"For verily I say unto you, That whosoever shall say unto this mountain, Be thou removed, and be thou cast into the sea; and shall not doubt in his heart, but shall believe that those things which he saith shall come to pass; he shall have whatsoever he saith" (Mark 11:23).

So when you speak to the mountain in prayer, you might pray:

Father, I come before You in Jesus' name and I speak to that mountain called menopause. I speak to my arteries and I command them to be normal, and I command them to be free of cholesterol plaque and fat buildup.

I command the calcium to remain within my bones and I say, "Bones, be strong and be strengthened with normal calcium levels." I speak to any mood changes, hot flashes, and sweats and command them to be gone in the name of Jesus.

I speak to the deep structures within my brain and command them to be protected from Alzheimer's disease and all forms of dementia and memory loss. I speak to my female organs and command them to be symptom-free, and I will not suffer the dryness and thinning effects from the lack of estrogen.

Thank You, Father, that my sleep will be peaceful, and I speak to my sleep and command it to remain normal.

Thank You, Father, for the power that You have given me through the name of Jesus to speak to my mountain. Thank You, Father, that through that authority I have dominion over the works of darkness that would attack my temple, which houses the precious treasure that You placed within me. In Jesus' name I pray. Amen.

PRINCIPLE 5:
PERSIST AND STAND FIRM IN YOUR PATHWAY

When you have a revelation of God's Pathway to Healing menopause in your life, stand firm in what He is guiding you to do. "Wherefore take unto you the whole armour of God, that ye may be able to withstand in the evil day, and having done all, to stand" (Ephesians 6:13).

The way you stand firm and persist is to follow a proper nutrition and supplement plan to maintain the correct balance of estrogen in your body, and you must persist in overcoming the annoying side effects as estrogen levels decrease, such as hot flashes and night sweats.

You must stand firm that as you do all you can do in the natural to protect your temple through nutrition, exercise, and the use of phytoestrogens, you will not suffer the ravages of blockage in the arteries, breast cancer, Alzheimer's disease, and so on.

PRINCIPLE 6:
MAINTAIN A FEISTY ATTITUDE
AGAINST THE WORKS OF DARKNESS

In order to persist and stand firm, you must shift to a different attitude. Avoid the danger of becoming passive, giving up, or failing to fight this battle. Be feisty — even violent — in your persistence. "And from the days of John the Baptist until now the kingdom of heaven suffereth violence, and the violent take it by force" (Matthew 11:12).

We encourage you to maintain a feisty attitude against all of the symptoms we have described that can take place in women's bodies with menopause. In other words, stand against damaged arteries, brittle bones, hot flashes, hair loss, and all symptoms which are works of the enemy.

In God's Pathway to Healing for women, He does not intend for menopause to be a time of misery; it is a time in which women should glow! The devil hates women because it was a woman who brought the Messiah, the Savior of the world, into our presence, and through Him we can be free of the devil's bondage and become God's child.

Remember that women were the first ones to arrive at the empty tomb and to rush back and proclaim the resurrection of Jesus Christ to men. (See Luke 24:6, 34.)

In the Garden of Eden (Genesis 3) the enemy attacked woman. She was tempted to sin and suffered later because of the attacks of the enemy. But through Jesus Christ, God has provided restoration for women. Through Jesus, women have a way to be loosed from not only the emotional and spiritual attacks of the enemy, but also the physical attacks of the enemy. Physical attacks like the uncomfortable and painful symptoms of menopause are not from God, but are attacks of the enemy, who seeks to hinder us from worshipping and serving the living God.

God has revealed a specific Pathway to Healing to keep women from suffering the ravages of menopause. He has a plan to protect women from both the annoying symptoms of the hot flashes and the sweats, and the rapid increase in diseases, such as heart disease, breast cancer, osteoporosis, and even Alzheimer's disease as the ovaries shut down after the childbearing years.

I believe the enemy attacks women for having gone through those childbearing years and producing offspring created in the image of God. So every time the enemy sees a baby created in God's image, his anger rises against women. He hates

God and all those created in His image who remind him of God.

However, God has created a Pathway to Healing menopause. He has provided a specific pathway for women to be protected: by natural estrogens. He put them in the plant kingdom to protect women from the attacks of the enemy in the natural realm.

Chapter 5

YOUR NEXT STEPS IN GOD'S PATHWAY TO HEALING

Chapter 5

YOUR NEXT STEPS
IN GOD'S PATHWAY
TO HEALING

You have begun an important journey in finding your Pathway to Healing menopause by reading this book and beginning to act upon the truths you have received.

We want to review and summarize for you the steps you need to take now as you receive God's unique Pathway to Healing for you.

Step 1. See your doctor. Consult a Christian physician or a competent medical doctor. We encourage you to find a

Christian doctor who will pray with you and give you all the facts known about your symptoms of menopause.

Step 2. Pray with understanding. Seek God in prayer and ask Him to reveal to you and to your doctor the best steps in the natural you can take in your Pathway to Healing.

Step 3. Ask the Holy Spirit to guide you to truth. For example, your doctor may advise you to use a medication like *Premarin*. Discuss with your physician the options of using *Menopause Support*. Explore all the aspects of the pathway we have shared with you, the pathway God has created to strengthen and guard your body. Allow the Holy Spirit to guide you to all truth.

Step 4. Maintain proper and healthy nutrition. Exercise and stay fit. We encourage you to stay on the Mediterranean diet and to use the foods, herbs, and supplements we discussed earlier to help your body overcome any painful symptoms of menopause.

Step 5. Stand firm in God's Pathway to Healing for you. Refuse to be discouraged or defeated. Be violently aggressive in prayer and in faith, claiming your healing in Jesus Christ.

We are praying that God will both reveal *His Pathway to Healing Menopause* to you and give you the strength and faith to walk in it.

REGINALD CHERRY, M.D.
A MEDICAL DOCTOR'S
TESTIMONY

The first six years of my life were lived in the dusty, rural town of Mansfield, in the Ouachita Mountains in western Arkansas. In those childhood years, I had one seemingly impossible dream — to be a doctor!

Through God's grace, I attended and graduated from Baylor University and The University of Texas Medical School in San Antonio, Texas. Throughout those years, I felt God tug on my heart a number of times, especially through Billy Graham as he preached on television. But I never surrendered my life to Jesus Christ.

In those early years of practicing medicine,

I met Dr. Kenneth Cooper and became trained in the field of preventive medicine. In the mid-seventies, I moved to Houston and established a medical practice for preventive medicine. Sadly, at that time money became a driving force in my life.

Nevertheless, God was so good to me. He brought into our clinic a nurse who became a Spirit-filled Christian, and she began praying for me. In fact, she had her whole church praying for me!

In my search for fulfillment and meaning in life, I called out to God one night in late November of 1979 and prayed, "Jesus, I give You everything I own. I'm sorry for the life I've lived. I want to live for You the rest of my days. I give You my life." A doctor had been born again. Oh, and by the way, that beautiful nurse who had prayed for me and shared Jesus with me is now my wife, Linda!

Not only did Jesus transform my life, He also transformed my medical practice. God spoke to me and said, "I want you to establish a Christian clinic. From now on when you practice medicine, you will be *ministering* to patients." I began to pray for patients seeking God's Pathway to Healing in the supernatural realm as well as in the natural realm.

Over the years, we have witnessed how God has miraculously used both supernatural and natural pathways to heal our patients and to demonstrate His marvelous healing and saving power.

I know what God has done in my life, and I know what God has done in the lives of our patients. He can do the same in your life! He has a unique Pathway to Healing for you! He is the Lord that heals you (see Exodus 15:26), and by His stripes you were healed (see Isaiah 53:5).

Know that Linda and I are standing with you as you seek *God's Pathway to Healing Menopause,* and as you walk in His Pathway to Healing for your life.

If you do not know Jesus Christ as your personal Lord and Savior, I invite you to pray this prayer and ask Jesus into your life:

> *Lord Jesus, I invite You into my life as my Lord and Savior. I repent of my past sins. I ask You to forgive me. Thank You for shedding Your blood on the cross to cleanse me from my sin and to heal me. I receive Your gift of everlasting life and surrender all to You. Thank You, Jesus, for saving me. Amen.*

Appendix

VITAMINS & ANTIOXIDANTS

In Matthew 24, Jesus describes several events that will occur in the last days. In Matthew 24:7, He specifically notes pestilences, or diseases. Many of the diseases we will see in the last days, AIDS for example, attack our immune system. We must, therefore, take measures to fortify and strengthen the immune system as much as possible.

Researchers have identified many substances that can strengthen the immune system and decrease the occurrence of many forms of cancer and heart disease. One such group is known as antioxidants. These include vitamin C, vitamin E, beta carotene, and selenium.

FOOD SOURCES OF ANTIOXIDANTS

Vitamin C: citrus fruits, strawberries, cantaloupe, broccoli, potatoes, tomatoes, and other fruits

Vitamin E: vegetable oils, wheat germ, whole grain bread, and pasta

Beta Carotene: broccoli, cantaloupe, carrots, spinach, squash, pumpkin, sweet potatoes, apricots, and other dark green, orange and yellow vegetables

Selenium: fish, meat, breads, and cereals

Another substance which seems to have a strong protective effect on numerous body functions is the trace mineral chromium. Found in brewer's yeast, whole wheat products, wheat bran, apple peel, and other substances, chromium plays a role in diabetes, cholesterol levels, heart disease, and cataracts. It also may be a significant deterrent to the aging process.

To insure an adequate intake of vitamins and minerals, many people take supplements. Based on current information, listed below are the supplements we personally take and those recommended by many researchers.

Supplement Dosages

Vitamin C	1,000 mg.	twice daily
Vitamin E	800 I.U.	once daily

Beta Carotene	15 mg.	once daily
Selenium	100 mcg.	twice daily
Chromium Picolinate	150 mcg.	twice daily
Coenzyme Q-10 (Co Q-10)	12.5 mg.	twice daily
B Complex Vitamins		daily
High Potency Multi Vitamin		daily
Calcium (carbonate, citrate, ascorbate)	1,000 mg.	once daily

Vitamin C should NOT be time-released, but take one in the a.m. and one in the p.m.

Vitamin E should be "natural."

Beta Carotene may come in 25,000 I.U., which is equal to 15 mg. NOTE: Smokers should not take this supplement.

High potency supplement, such as *Basic Nutrient Support.*

NOTE: TAKE VITAMINS WITH A MEAL.

CHILDREN: Above recommendations are for adults and children above the age if 16. Children ages 16 and under should use a multi-purpose vitamin such as "Flintstones," etc.

RESOURCES AVAILABLE FROM DR. CHERRY MINISTRIES

The Doctor and the Word and *The Bible Cure* — Discover God's Pathway to Healing for your life and how to apply His Bible cure in prayer and healthy nutrition. A ministry donation of $27.

Pathway to Healing Seminar — 8 audio tapes filled with life-changing revelation on God's healing pathway for your life. $29.99 ministry donation.

Bound volume of Dr. Cherry's *Study Guides* from his popular Trinity Broadcasting Network (TBN) program, "The Doctor and the Word." $20 donation.

Order *Menopause Support* — $25.95 for a month's supply by calling toll-free:

1-800-339-5952

BECOME A PATHWAY TO HEALING PARTNER

Dr. Cherry is viewed on TBN and other television stations throughout America weekly. You can become a part of this vital ministry and also receive a special subscription to the *Pathway to Healing* magazine which is mailed as a gift to Dr. Cherry's ministry partners.

In this exciting, magazine, you will read about the latest medical breakthroughs and discover exciting information and insights in these features:

Fearfully and Wonderfully Made — Uncovers how God made our bodies to resist disease.

Menopause Support—Dr. Cherry has formulated a unique natural supplement to help bring balance and protection to this challenging time in a woman's life. *Menopause Support* is based on his 25 years of research and medical practice. It's a combination of 7 minerals, herbs, plant extracts, and enzymes—everything Dr. Cherry recommends specifically to help women stay comfortable and full of life during and after menopause. Menopause Support helps promote hormonal balance, increased energy, strong bones, and healthy cells. Best when used with *Basic Nutrient Support.* Call **1-800-339-5952** for information and ordering. Mention Service Code **K184.** Online, visit www.AbundantNutrition.com

$25.95 + S&H

ABOUT THE AUTHORS

Reginald B. Cherry, M.D., did his premed at Baylor University, graduated from the University of Texas Medical School, and practiced diagnostic and preventive medicine for over 25 years. His work in medicine has been recognized and honored by the city of Houston and by the governor of Texas, George W. Bush. Dr. Cherry's wife, Linda, is a clinical nurse and has assisted Dr. Cherry in seeing patients for the past 25 years. Dr. Cherry and Linda also appear weekly on their television program, "The Doctor and the Word," which goes into over 100 million households. Dr. Cherry speaks and lectures extensively, and his first two books, *The Doctor and the Word* and *The Bible Cure*, each have made the best sellers' list.

Become a Pathway Partner today by calling toll-free:

1-888-DrCherry

(1-888-372-4377)

Or writing:

Reginald B. Cherry Ministries

P.O. Box 27711

Houston, TX 77227